Your Body, Sick and Well:
How Do You Know?

The Poemenclature Series

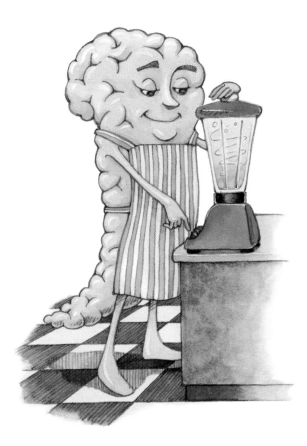

Praise for
Your Body Sick and Well: How Do You Know?

"Your Body Sick and Well: How Do You Know? is a perfect introduction into the complex world of organs, disease, and the tools needed for diagnosing and treating many serious childhood conditions. Using playful poems and "Learn More!" sections on each page, Dr. Cunningham breaks down these topics in a way that children and their parents alike can understand. Susan Detwiler's charming and clever illustrations further enhance and explain the text in ways that children can relate to. As a former neo-natal and pediatric nurse, now children's book author and illustrator as well as mom to three children, I believe this book in *The Poemenclature Series* would make an excellent addition and resource for school classrooms and doctor offices, and I recommend it to any parent looking for books to explain these serious topics in a very child-friendly way."

— Joan Waites, recipient of the Teacher's Choice Award and the Benjamin Franklin Award, and illustrator of many popular children's books, including *What's New at the Zoo? An Animal Adding Adventure* (2009)

"Dr. Steven Cunningham's new book of poems about the human body is loaded with humor, facts, and fancy, along with some whimsical color illustrations by Susan Detwiler. In addition to human anatomy, the poems reference diseases and doctor's tools. Enjoy it!"

— Douglas Florian, author of *Dinothesaurus* (2009), a Kirkus Reviews Best Book of the Year, a Horn Book Fanfare List selection and a Junior Library Guild selection; *Lizards, Frogs and Polliwogs* (2005), a Bulletin Blue Ribbon Book; and *Bow Wow Meow Meow* (2003), Gryphon Award-winner and *Parents* magazine Best Book of the Year

"This is an exciting and worthwhile addition to literature for kids. The poems are fun to read and convey a lot of information. The "Learn More!" section on each topic is wonderful. The illustrations are lively, accurate, and often amusing."

— Sue Poduska, creator of GradeReading.net, a suite of blogs that reviews children's literature

Your Body, Sick and Well:
How Do You Know?

The Poemenclature Series

Steven Clark Cunningham, M.D.

Illustrations by Susan Detwiler

Three Conditions Press
Baltimore, MD

Revised and Republished by Three Conditions Press (2019), Baltimore, MD.
An initial version of this book appeared under the title *Poemenclature: Poems About Your Body*
in Great Britain and the United States by Under the Maple Tree Books,
an imprint of Knox Robinson Publishing (2017).

ISBN: 978-0-9721241-7-1

Library of Congress Cataloging-in-Publication Data:
Library of Congress Control Number: 2019911633

Book Design: Deb Dulin
Editing: Rosemary Klein
Special Thanks to: Shayna Blank, Douglas Florian, and Myriam Gorospe

Visit https://stevenclarkcunningham.net

To Rosemary Klein, whose friendship and care with language have been for these past 20+ years so inspiring and sustaining to my work.

"A main source of our failure to understand is that we do not command
a clear view of the use of our words."

Ludwig Wittgenstein, an elementary-school teacher for six years,
and one of the greatest philosophers of the twentieth century, who spent much
of his life studying how we use language

"If names be incorrect, language is not in accordance
with the truth of things."

Confucius, a philosopher from ancient China and that country's first private teacher,
who was quite strict about knowing the meaning of words and using them correctly

"Call him Voldemort, Harry. Always use the proper name for things."

Albus Dumbledore, Headmaster of Hogwarts School of Witchcraft and Wizardry,
in *Harry Potter and the Sorcerer's Stone*, by J. K. Rowling

Contents

Preface: Inventing a Word

In a word, it is a lot of *fun* — and pretty meaningful — to invent a word yourself. But what in the world does "poemenclature" mean (and why did I invent it)???

When you play *with* words, sometimes you combine them and come up with a new word. Then you have a play *on* words, often one that is very funny. For example: What do you get when you cross a snake and a pie? A pie-thon, of course!

"Poemenclature," the play on the words that I introduce in this book, combines two words: "nomenclature" and "poems."

"Nomenclature" is about naming things. And "poems" are, of course, collections of words that often have rhythm, and sometimes rhyme, and try to make you see things in a different way than you might otherwise.

Soooo, poems such as the ones in this book (and in my last book *Dinosaur Name Poems*) allow me to define the names of things to help you learn about and understand them. I hope you enjoy saying the word I invented. And I hope you enjoy reading the poems (out loud is especially fun) in this book!

Oh, and by the way, while you are reading this book, notice that some words in the "Learn More!" sections are **boldfaced and italicized**. This is to tell you that these words, which you may or may not already know, are defined in the glossary at the back of the book.

Dictionaries and encyclopedias can give you much, much more about the meaning and use of the word "nomenclature," as well as all words in this book and everywhere. Check them out!

*PS: Speaking of calling things by their right names, I think that's really important. After all, how **can** we talk about things, if we don't know their names??? That's why I totally agree with what Confucius, Wittgenstein, and Dumbledore say in the epigraphs a few pages back!*

Part One:

Anatomy
(Organ Names)

Heart

300 liters per hour
Is the blood-pumping power
Of the human heart,
Which feeds your brain
To make you smart
Enough to paint a flower.

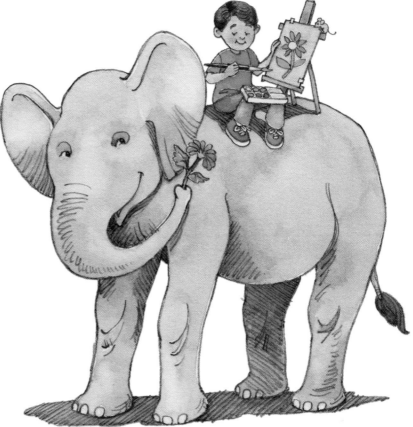

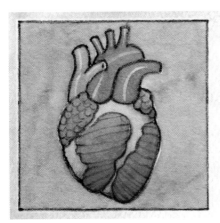

LEARN MORE! Your heart is a muscular pump made up of four compartments, or chambers (two *atria* and two *ventricles*). It is about the size of your fist. As you get bigger so does your heart, and it slows down. A baby's resting heart rate is 120 beats per minute. A 7-year-old's is 90 beats per minute, while an adult's heart beats about 70 times per minute. A mouse's heart beats 600 times per minute but an elephant's heart only 30 beats per minute.

Brain

How many nerve cells live in the brain?
If you are a little worm it's 302,
But it's 100 billion if you happen to be you.

1 000 000   one million
1 000 000 000   one billion
100 000 000 000   one hundred billion

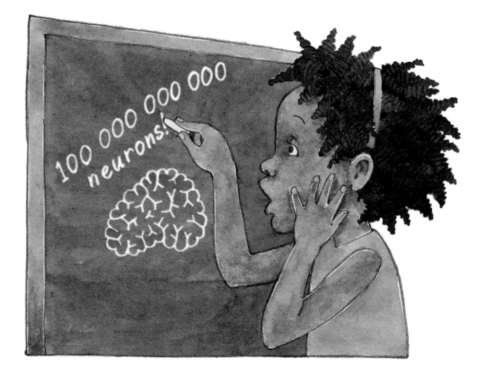

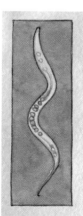 **LEARN MORE!** *C. elegans* is a certain kind of soil worm, called a nematode, that lives all over the world. It is only one milimeter (about 1/32 of an inch) long, has a life cycle of only three weeks, and its brain has only 302 **neurons**, or **nerve cells**. The human brain, on the other hand, has about 100 billion **neurons**! To get an idea for how much that is, just consider how much one billion is: To count to a billion would take you 30 years counting nonstop! A billion minutes ago was almost 2000 years ago! A billion hours ago was the Stone Age! A billion months ago, dinosaurs walked the earth! Now, if you think a billion is a lot, just use some of your **neurons** to consider that there are 100 times that many **neurons** in your brain, so use them!

Blood

It's red, it's in your head.
It's in your toes and elbows.
Wherever there is some of you,
There too it goes.
Everywhere, except nails and hair,
It carries your air.
(Really! There's air in there!)
In no one place for long it dwells.
It's always moving round and round your cells.

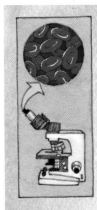

LEARN MORE! The "*air*" that your blood carries is mostly oxygen and carbon dioxide. Blood carries fresh inhaled oxygen (O_2) from your lungs to your cells and carries carbon dioxide (CO_2) waste from your *cells* to your lungs to be exhaled. These *gases* (oxygen and carbon dioxide) are carried by your blood in two main ways: One way is attached to protein called *hemoglobin* in *red blood cells*, which under a microscope look like little dimpled discs. The other way is dissolved in liquid blood like the way carbon dioxide is dissolved in carbonated beverages or like the way air is dissolved in fish-tank water (the reason air is bubbled through tank water is to dissolve oxygen in the water for the fish to "breathe").

Pancreas:
A Two-for-One Organ

Your pancreas makes insulin,
Which helps get sugar into you.
This should make you happy, make you grin.
But that's not all this organ can do!

Insulin's very important – that's true –
But so is the juice your pancreas makes:
A juice that takes all food that you chew –
Meats like steaks and treats like cakes –

And into smaller and smaller pieces it breaks
Every drop of spinach-asparagus-sauerkraut soup.
Yes, without this gland you'd have belly aches,
And lack of sugar would make you stoop and droop;
You would be completely pooped!

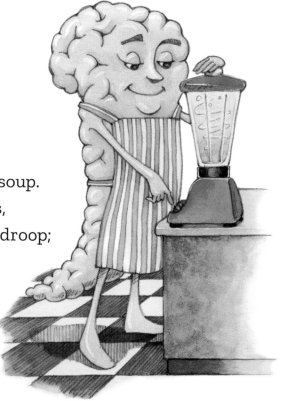

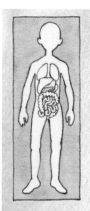

LEARN MORE! Even though it looks like just one organ on the outside, the pancreas (my favorite organ) is really two **organs** rolled into one: One "organ" is an **exocrine** (EX-o-crin) gland and the other organ an **endocrine** (EN-do-crin) gland. The **exocrine cells** of the pancreas secrete digestive enzymes into the intestine that help to break down your food into useful parts that can be absorbed by your intestines into your bloodstream. The **endocrine cells** of the pancreas secrete **hormones** like **insulin** directly into your bloodstream to help your body use sugar, which is the main fuel supply for your brain!

Intestines

Everything you eat,
Every pickled beet,
And every candied treat,
Every mouthful of rice, corn, oats, and wheat,
All the veggies and all the meat,
Travels your gut for 20 feet!

What happens inside is really kind of neat:
As food moves from your mouth towards your feet,
Your small intestine takes fuel to make heat
(And more of you – That's no small feat!),
Your large intestine takes back water,
While the rest you just excrete!

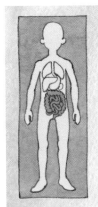

LEARN MORE! The "small" intestine is not so small. It's actually quite long (over 20 feet). And the surface area is even more impressive: If the lining of the intestinal tract were smooth and flat, the surface area would be less than 10 square feet, but it's really almost 10,000 square feet, or about the size of a baseball field. Why? Because the lining is not smooth and flat, but has folds that increase the area by about 3x. Each fold has microscopic, fingerlike folds called *villi* that increase the area another 10x. Each of these *villi* have *cells* with even smaller *microvilli* that increase the area by approximately another 20x (10 square feet x 3 x 10 x 20 = 9,000). You've got a lot of guts!

Lungs

They are filled with fluid at first,
Then you're born and breathe a burst
Of cold, and then the fluid goes out
While air rushes in and lets you shout.

And thus they let you
Exhale CO2 and inhale O2
In and out, starting on day one,
Again and again, until your setting sun.

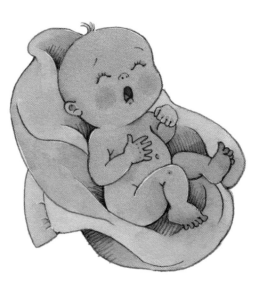

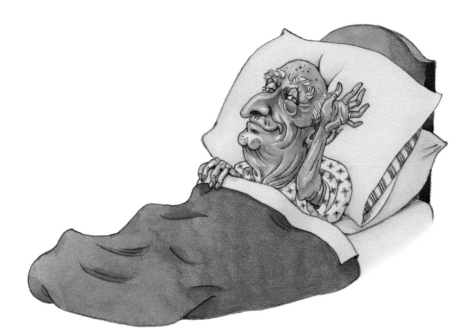

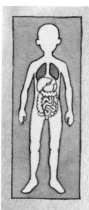 **LEARN MORE!** Before you are born (when you are still a *fetus* inside your mother), blood mostly bypasses your lungs, since they are not inflated and cannot provide oxygen from the air. Instead, the mother's lungs provide the oxygen, which reaches the baby through the *placenta* and the *umbilical cord*. From there the oxygen-rich blood bypasses the lungs and goes straight to the heart to be pumped around the body to give all the baby's *cells* oxygen. At birth, a major change in blood flow happens: When the baby takes its first gasping breath, oxygen-rich air rushes in and the lungs expand. They are then suddenly supplied with blood to exchange oxygen and carbon dioxide so that the baby can breathe like the rest of us!

Bones

A person's bones,
Much more than telephones,
Shiny stones, or brass trombones
(Even pistachio ice-cream cones),
Are one of the most useful things
That a person owns.

Without your bones,
You couldn't answer that phone,
Hold that stone, trom that bone,
Or lick or nibble that ice cream cone!
And your blood and calcium would have
No place to call home!

LEARN MORE! Your bones (all 206 of them!) have many useful functions. They protect, move, and support the soft *organs* of the body, they produce *red blood cells* and *white blood cells*, and they store minerals like calcium.

Liver

Even though
Just a sliver of your liver
Can do the whole organ's work
(Producing protein,
Busting out bile,
Metabolizing molecules),
What's best is that if you cut out the rest,
Say, for example, eight parts of ten,
Those eight parts grow right back again!

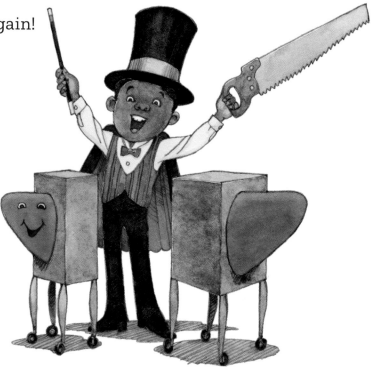

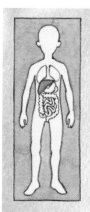

LEARN MORE! The liver (my second-favorite organ) is the only organ that has such a tremendous ability to regenerate itself. Sometimes, because of **tumors**, infections, or injuries, a surgeon may have to **resect** part of the liver. Eighty percent of an otherwise healthy liver may by safely removed with no major change in liver function. What's more amazing is that from the remaining 20%, all or most of the missing 80% will grow back again, much like the remaining branches of a tree or bush will get larger after being pruned (cut back). The main functions of the liver are to produce a wide variety of proteins that perform important bodily functions, to make the bile that helps to digest food, and to **metabolize** chemicals, medicines, and other **molecules**.

Keeping the Inside in, the Skin

Some is thick, some is thin,
It covers your shin, it covers your chin,
And all of the shins and chins of all of your kin.

Some is dark, some is light,
Some is red, blue or white,
Some is thick and bumpy, some is slight,
The skin that you have, for you is just right!

Some is bare and some sprouts hair
(Mostly just on top),
But some has hair everywhere.

The most important thing I'll tell you about
Is that your skin is how you win
The battle to keep the outside out
And the inside in.

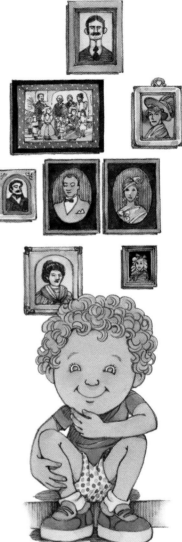

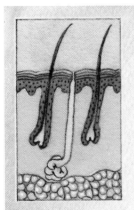

LEARN MORE! Your skin is your largest *organ*. One of its most important functions is to keep your clean, wet inside *organs* safe from the dirty, dry outside world that would make you sick if it weren't for your skin. Your skin renews itself completely every month or so. One of the main characteristics of human skin is the presence of hair follicles, which all mammals have.

Your Cleaning Bean, the Spleen

Yes,
Your
Spleen
Looks
Like
A
Mis-
Shapen
Bean
!!!

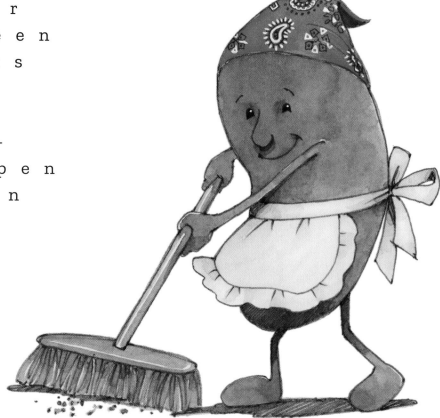

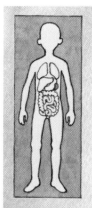

LEARN MORE! Your spleen is very important early in your life, when it makes blood *cells*, prevents infections, and cleans your blood. Later in life it becomes less important and joins rank with the *appendix* and *gallbladder* in the list of organs you don't really need to live a happy and healthy life.

Stomach

The stomach is what
Lives between the gullet and gut.
As you might guess,
Its job is to digest.

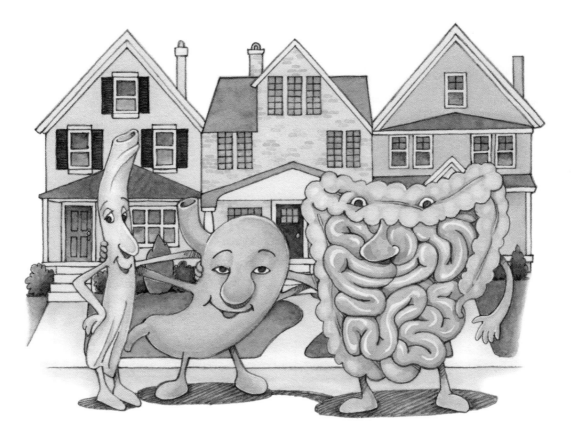

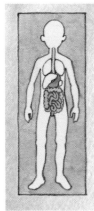

LEARN MORE! The stomach not only helps to begin to digest your food but also makes *hormones* and stores the food, which it releases slowly into the intestines, where most of digestion happens. Usually what we call a "stomach ache" is not from the stomach at all but from some other abdominal *organ* like the intestines. And, by the way, the "gullet" and the "gut" are everyday terms (also called lay terms) for the esophagus and the intestines, respectively.

Kidneys, Kid Knees, and Squid Knees

Every kid has a kidney or two.
Most are neatly shaped like beans,
But some are connected like a horseshoe!

"Don't kid me about my kidney!" you say,
"A horseshoe kidney – that can't be!"
But I wouldn't kid you: it's true!

Horseshoe or bean, kid, horse, squid or shrew,
The kidney cleans the blood and makes you pee.

In addition to kidneys most every kid has kid knees, too
(Almost always, of those there also are two).

And, while every squid also has kidneys,
To help *them* make *their* pee pees,
Not a single squid,
Not even a kid squid,
Has squid knees!

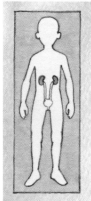

LEARN MORE! The kidneys filter or clean over 1000 liters of blood per day and make about 1-1.5 liters of urine per day. This is a very useful function, but they also produce *hormones* that are important because they regulate the balance of salts in the blood and help control blood pressure.

Part Two:

Pathology
(Disease Names)

Diabetes Mellitus
(DIE-ah-BEE-tees MEL-i-tis)

"A honey-sweet passer through"
dia- across, through + *-bainein* to walk, go; *mellitus* honey

If you have diabetes,
Don't be too greedies
With the treaties.

If you don't have diabetes,
The same is true for you, Sweeties,

Because if you're greedies
With the treaties,

You'll rot your teethies,
And feel yucky from your head to your feeties.

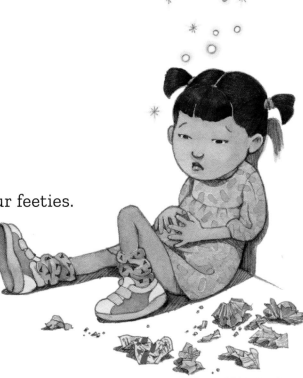

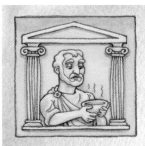 **LEARN MORE!** Diabetes Mellitus, a disease in which the body's inability to produce enough *insulin*, or to use the *insulin* well, causes elevated glucose (sugar) levels in the blood. It was first described by an ancient Greek physician (Aretaeus), who coined the term *diabetes* because of the large amount of urine that diabetics have "go through" them. The term *mellitus* was added later because of the sweet taste (that's right, taste) of the urine, which is due to the large amount of sugar that the urine contains.

Congenital Cardiac Defect
(CON-jen-i-tul CARD-ee-ack DEE-fect)

"Born-with heart defect"
con- together, with + *-genitus* born; cardio- heart;
defectus defect, want

I was born with a broken heart:
Called congenital cardiac defect.

When I was a baby they took it apart,
Then the parts had to reconnect,
Then they had to restart my heart!

They sent me home, where I now reflect
Upon the way this made me smart:
Because now when my toys get wrecked,
I give thanks that it isn't my heart.

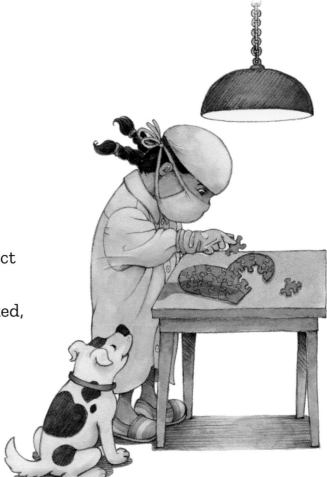

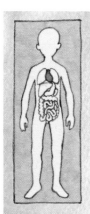

LEARN MORE! There are many different kinds of congenital heart defects. Nearly all of them cause problems with blood flow through the heart: either that the flow is partially blocked or that it flows in an abnormal pattern. The most common is called a ventricular septal defect, or VSD for short. In this congenital heart defect, there is an opening in the wall that is supposed to completely separate the two **ventricles**. Such an opening can also occur in the wall that is supposed to separate the two **atria**, and that is called an atrial septal defect, or ASD.

Meningitis
(MEN-inj-eye-tis)

"Membrane swelling or inflammation"
Meningae- membrane or lining + *-itis* inflammation

The cover of brain
Is smooth and slick,
But when the lining is sick
It gets rough and thick!

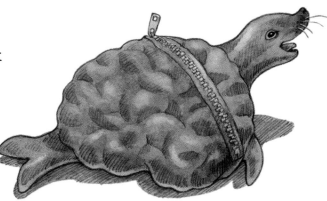

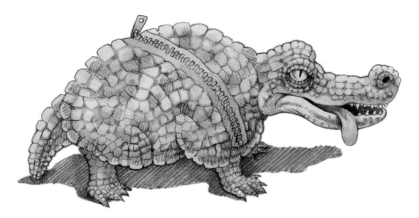

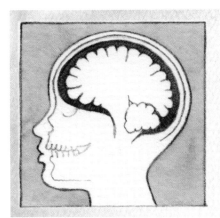

LEARN MORE! The meninges (men-INJ-eez) is the lining of the brain and spinal cord and is made up of three separate layers, an outer layer called the dura mater (DER-ah MAH-ter), a middle layer called the arachnoid (ah-RAK-noyd) membrane, and an inner layer called the pia mater (PEE-ah MAH-ter). *Inflammation* of this lining is called meningitis and is often caused by bacteria or viruses. Meningitis can be mild or life-threatening.

Colitis

(COL-eye-tis)

"Colon swelling or inflammation"
colo- colon + *-itis* inflammation

When your colon is inflamed
And cannot by diet or drugs be tamed,
You cannot be blamed
When it seems like always
To the loo for another poo
You are aimed.

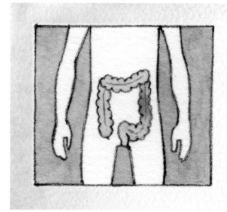

LEARN MORE! Colitis is ***inflammation*** of the colon. It can be caused by certain ***bacteria***, ***viruses***, drugs, immune system malfunction, or other factors. One of the most important jobs of the colon is to absorb water (so that your poo comes out solid). Therefore, when the colon is ***inflamed***, it doesn't do a good job absorbing water and this usually results in diarrhea.

Fracture
(FRACT-er)

"a break or to break,"
fractura break

A fracture is a break
(As in a broken arm),

A tough break, a major ache,
Can hurt so much as to make
You quake and shake,
(And can cause great harm),

Can keep you awake at night
And take the delight out of baking a cake
Or walking around your favorite lake
(Or through your favorite farm).

So beware – make no mistake –
It can happen anywhere
(With or without your lucky charm):

You could break your arm
Unless, of course, you happen to be a snake!

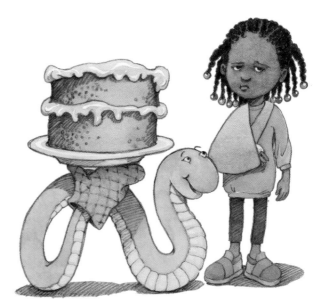

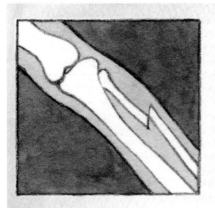

LEARN MORE! Fractures are categorized into two main kinds: 1) simple, or closed, fractures in which the overlying skin is intact and 2) compound, or open, fractures in which the fractured bones are exposed to the outside world through a skin wound associated with the fracture.

Cancer
(CAN-ser)

"Cancer"
karkinos crab

Cancer keeps on growing
When normal parts are slowing.
The really hard part is knowing
How to keep on going,
To keep your smile showing,
When the cancer keeps on growing.

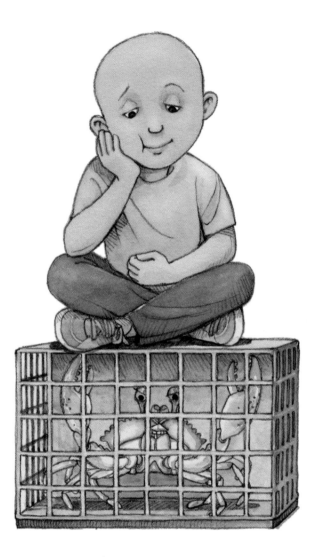

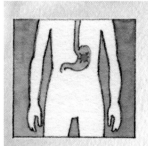

LEARN MORE! Our bodies are made up of trillions of tiny building blocks, called *cells*. Normally, *cells* grow when they are supposed to, like when there is an injury that needs to heal, and they stop when healing is done. Your body does this by sending signals to tell the *cells* when to grow and when to stop. In *cancer*, one *cell* loses the ability to respond to these signals and begins to grow out of control. The reason that *cancer* is named after the crab is because when ancient Greek physicians first saw a *cancer* in the stomach of a patient, they noticed that the overgrowing tumor had big blood vessels going to and from it all around and it reminded them of the way legs extend out from the body of a crab.

Leukemia
(loo-KEY-mee-ah)

"White blood"
leuko- white + *-emia* blood

White blood cells,
Like chocolate bells,
Pasta shells,
Flowery smells,
And hair gels,
Are good when just
The right number dwells.

But when there are too many,
Or too much of any of these,
The body yells
That trouble
Is what that spells.

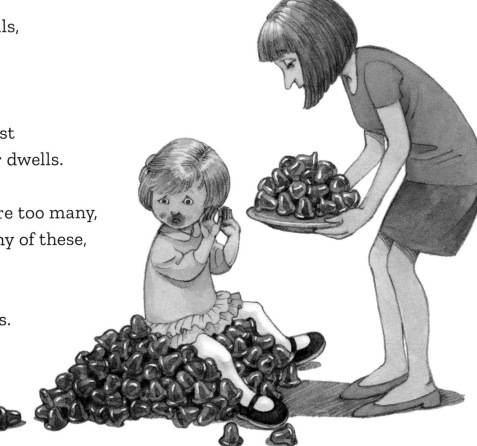

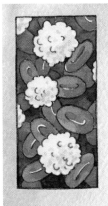

LEARN MORE! Leukemia is the most common *cancer* of childhood. *Cancers* can arise from most any normal *cell* in the body. Our bodies contain about 200 different *cell* types, including white and red blood *cells*. *White blood cells* are germ-fighters and you could not live without them. Like many things in life, such as chocolate bells and pasta shells, the right amount is good but too much could be bad. It is good to know that sometimes the right amount of something is simply yummy or may even be life-saving, and sometimes too much can be just yucky or may even be life-threatening.

Part Three:

Instruments
(Tool Names)

Stethoscope
(STEH-thuh-scope)

"Chest-looker"
stethos- chest + *-skopein* to look at, examine

You may listen to my chest.
I promise I'll do my best,
To breathe in deep
And to keep
Very still
As your stethoscope
Checks my heart
And my lungs
(Oh! Here it comes,
Not *too* icy-cold I hope!)
You will listen and know
So much about my heart flow
As long as I am still, yes Sir,
And as long as your hands
Aren't also...

    ....BBBRRRrrr!

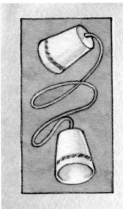

LEARN MORE! The first stethoscope was invented by a French physician named René Laennec. This was a simple *monaural* device with two ends, one held to the patient's chest and one to the physician's ear. This first stethoscope and modern stethoscopes work like a toy string telephone: sound vibrations are transmitted from the source (a person's voice in a string telephone or your heart beating in your chest) and they travel along the string or the tube to the listener's ear. Have you ever made a string telephone? Just cut a hole in the bottom of two paper cups, and attach them with a string like in the picture (knot the two ends to keep the string in the cups). Give it a try!

Thermometer
(ther-MOM-eh-ter)

"Heat-measurer"
 therm- heat + *-metron* measure

Tickly in my ear,
Icicle-ly under my arm,
Sticky on my forehead,
And under my tongue,
    awfully teeth-clinky,
It can measure my heat
Everywhere, it seems,
Except under my feet.

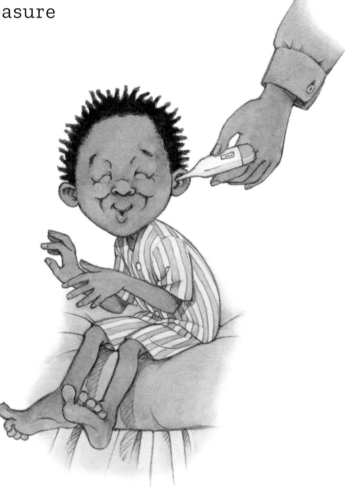

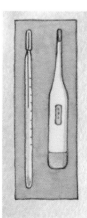

LEARN MORE! Two common thermometers are *liquid* (or bulb) and spring thermometers. They both work on the principle that **matter** expands (gets larger) when heated and contracts (gets smaller) when cooled. In *liquid* ones, a small drop of a heat-sensitive *liquid* fills a bulb at the bottom of a long, very thin, hollow tube. As the *liquid* (mercury in older gray ones or colored alcohol in newer red ones) warms, it expands to fill the tube marked with numbers for the temperature. In spring thermometers, a heat-sensitive metal spring is attached to a pointer on a numbered circle, and as the metal expands or contracts the pointer moves around the circle. Some newer thermometers use crystals that change colors.

Sphygmomanometer
(sfig-moh-mah-NAH-meh-ter)

"Pulse-pressure-measurer"
sphygmos- pulse + *-mano-* gas + *-metron* measure

A sphygmo-what-er?

A sphygmo-man-on-the-myrrh?

A sphyg-mommy-waiter?

A sphyg-no-manowar-eater?

A sphyg-more-many-more-than-her?

A sphyg-oh-what-ever!

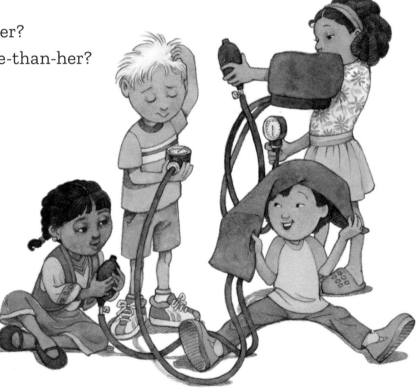

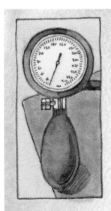

LEARN MORE! A sphygmomanometer is an ***instrument*** used to measure blood pressure. It is basically just a balloon that is wrapped around your arm and inflated to a pressure higher than your blood pressure. This stops the flow of blood in your arm for a few moments until the cuff is deflated. As the balloon slowly deflates, the pressure it applies to your arm decreases until blood flow returns. At that point the blood flow is detected by a machine or by the person listening to your blood vessel with a stethoscope (you can actually hear it flow). Blood pressure is measured at two points in the heart cycle, once at ***systole*** (a heartbeat, when the pressure is highest) and once at ***diastole*** (between beats, when the pressure is lowest).

Chemotherapy
(KEY-mo-THER-a-pee)

"Chemical healing"
  chemo- chemicals or drugs + *-therapia* healing, treatment

I have cancer,
And chemo's
An answer.

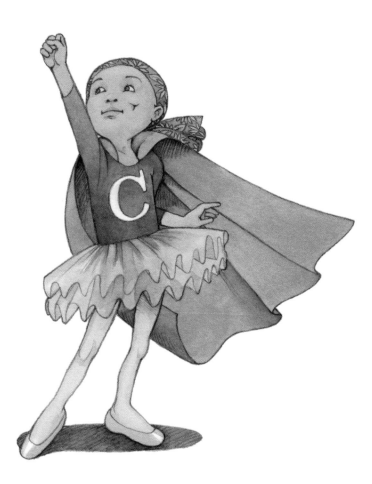

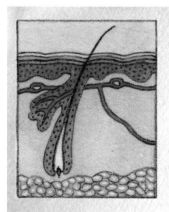

LEARN MORE! Chemotherapy is often given to patients who have **cancer**. Many chemotherapy medicines act by killing fast-growing **cells** such as cancer **cells**. These medicines also tend to kill some normal **cells**, especially those that also grow fast, such as hair follicles and intestinal **cells**. That's why sometimes people taking chemotherapy lose their hair or feel nauseated.

Radiology
(RAY-dee-ALL-oh-gee)

"Radiation science"
radio- radiation + *-ology* science, discipline, study, discourse

Radiology is where you go
When the doctors want to know
What's hiding down below.

On top they can see your skin,
But what they do in Radiology
Is have an X-ray look within.

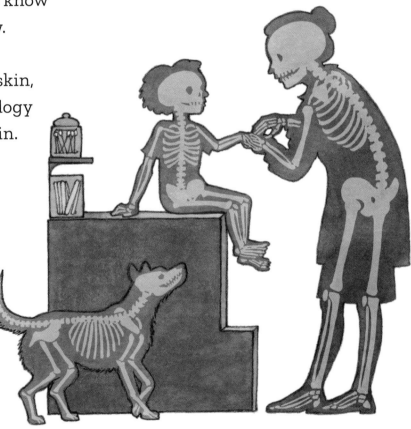

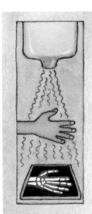

LEARN MORE! Radiation and its medical uses are studied and used in the science of radiology. It's also the name of the department in the hospital where radiology tests (like X-rays) are performed. X-rays are one of many forms of radiation (other forms are microwaves, radio waves, and light). All X-ray tests, such as chest X-rays, X-rays of arms and legs, and CAT scans (which also use X-rays), are able to give a picture because hard, dense structures like bone block the X-rays while soft things, such as skin, fat, and air, let them pass right through. Just like the sun's rays cast shadows, so do the X-rays, and the "shadows" of the X-rays are captured on film for the doctors to look at.

Anesthesia
(AN-es-thee-zjha)

"Without sensation"
an- without + *-aisthesis* sensation

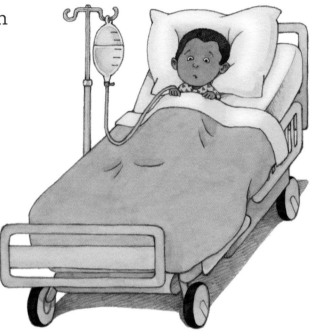

An operation is what I need
And I am terribly afraid:
Will it hurt? Will I bleed?
And what about that scalpel blade?

The doctors have come and gone again,
Have told me all about it,
Have done their best to explain,
But I still don't really get it:

This mask smells funny. Will I suffer?
How will I know once it's begun?
Oh, I wish I could be tougher!
What's that you say?!? It's already done?!?

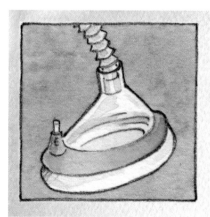

LEARN MORE! Before operations, anesthesiologists give medicines to induce, or cause, anesthesia, which is insensitivity to pain. In addition, some of the medicines anesthesiologists give before and during an operation cause *amnesia*.

32

Glossary

Air: the stuff you breathe: mostly nitrogen (about 78%), partly oxygen (about 21%), and a tiny amount of other gases (such as argon and carbon dioxide).

Amnesia: loss of memory, generally severe.

Anatomy: the study of the structure of **organisms**.

Appendix: a small tube that is closed at one end and projects out from the first part of the **colon**, in the lower right side of the abdomen.

Artery: a blood vessel that carries fresh blood (with oxygen from the lungs) away from the heart to the other organs. Compare with **vein**.

Atrium: one of the two small, upper, less muscular chambers of the heart that receives blood from the **veins** of the body and pumps blood to the **ventricle** of the same side (right or left).

Bacteria: single-celled microscopic organisms that live in soil, water, and the bodies of plants and animals (including yours!). They are important because they are required for good health but can also cause diseases.

Bile: a thick, bitter, yellow-reddish fluid that is secreted by the liver, stored and concentrated in the **gallbladder**, and from there released into the small intestine when you eat, to help to digest and absorb food, especially fats.

Cancer: a disease in which **tumors** grow uncontrolled. They can spread by invading nearby structures. They can also spread to other parts of the body (can metastasize). Cancers can be liquid, like leukemia, or solid, like brain cancer.

Cells: the building blocks of all living **organisms**. All of your organs are made up of cells.

Diastole: the relaxation of the heart by which the heart fills in preparation for another contraction (**systole**) to pump blood forward. Compare with **systole**.

Endocrine: secreting internally (directly into the bloodstream). Examples of endocrine glands include the thyroid gland (in the neck), testicles and ovaries, and the endocrine pancreas gland. These glands secrete **hormones** that help keep your body in good working order.

Exocrine: secreting externally (not into the blood, but instead into the outside world, or into the ducts or the gastrointestinal tract, that lead to the outside world). Examples of exocrine glands include sweat glands, salivary (spit) glands, mammary (breast) glands, and the exocrine pancreas gland.

Fetus: what we call a baby before the baby is born. In other words, an unborn human being, especially from two months of pregnancy until birth (before two months, it's called an embryo).

Gallbladder: a muscular sac attached to the liver. It stores and concentrates bile from the liver. When you eat, bile is released from the gallbladder into the small intestines to help you digest your food, especially fatty foods. Compare with *bile*.

Gas: see *matter*.

Hemoglobin: the protein in *red blood cells* that transports oxygen and carbon dioxide.

Hormone: a substance that living *cells* produce and secrete into the bloodstream, usually traveling to a distant part of the body to perform some specific function, for example processing sugar, digesting food, or controlling blood pressure.

Inflammation: your body's response to injured *cells*. All the tiny blood vessels in an inflamed area dilate (enlarge) and then the nearby cells release signals that cause *white blood cells* to come in and start cleaning up the infection or contamination. As the white blood cells do their work, they cause the typical symptoms of inflammation: redness, swelling, warmth, pain, and sometimes fever.

Instrument: a tool or device used to achieve something.

Insulin: a *hormone* secreted by the *endocrine* pancreas that is essential for helping your body to use sugar properly.

Liquid: see *matter*.

Matter: the substance of which a physical object is composed or made. There are three main types of matter here on earth: *gases*, *liquids*, and *solids*. A *gas* is a fluid form of matter that has no independent shape, is completely elastic, and expands indefinitely. A *liquid* is also a fluid form of matter that also has no independent shape, but is not very elastic (cannot be easily compressed, or squeezed, to a smaller size, like a *gas* can), and does not expand indefinitely. A *solid* is a form of matter that does have an independent shape and does not flow (at least not fast enough for you to notice) but rather keeps its shape.

Metabolism: the processes by which complex substances in our *cells* are built up or broken down to maintain life.

Metabolize: to break down by *metabolism*.

Microvilli: tiny fingerlike structures that line the **cells** that make up **villi**, and further help to absorb digested food.

Molecule: the smallest particle of a substance having all the characteristics of that substance.

Monaural: hearing with or involving only one ear.

Nerve: another word for a **neuron**.

Neuron: a fiber-like **cell** that receives signals (nerve impulses), decides on their importance, and then sends the signals to another neuron or an organ. Neurons make up the brain, the spinal canal, and extend to all parts of the body. Sensory neurons send signals from the body to the brain and motor neurons send signals from the brain to the body, allowing all parts of the body to communicate with each other.

Organ: a structure consisting of **cells** and **tissues** performing some specific function in an **organism**.

Organism: an individual able to carry on the activities of life through its **organs** that have separate functions but are dependent on each other. A living being is an organism.

Pathology: the study of diseases.

Placenta: the organ connecting the **umbilical cord** of the **fetus** to the mother (to her uterus, or womb, which is where the **fetus** lives until birth).

Proteins: substances that consist of chains of **molecules** called amino acids. They are essential for life and are supplied by various foods, such as meat, milk, eggs, nuts, and beans.

Red blood cells: blood cells that contain **hemoglobin**, which binds and carries oxygen and carbon dioxide back and forth between the lungs and the other organs.

Resect: to cut out, to perform a **resection** (the surgical removal of part or all of an **organ** or structure).

Scalpel: a small, straight, thin-bladed, knife used especially in surgery.

Solid: see **matter**.

Systole: the contraction of the heart by which blood is forced forward in circulation. Compare with **diastole**.

Tissue: a collection of **cells** and the substance between them, which forms the basic structures of the body in an **organism**.

Tumor: an abnormal, uncontrolled growth of tissue.

Umbilical cord: a cord connecting a *fetus'* navel (belly button) to its *placenta*.

Vein: a blood vessel that carries used blood (with carbon dioxide waste) to the heart to get pumped to the lungs. In the lungs, the carbon dioxide is exchanged for new oxygen for the heart to pump to the other organs again. Compare with *artery*.

Ventricle: one of the two large, lower, more muscular chambers of the heart that receives blood from the **atrium** of the same side (right or left) and then pumps the blood into the **arteries**.

Villi: small fingerlike structures that line the small intestines and help to absorb digested food.

Virus: any of a large group of very tiny infectious agents that are too small to be seen with an ordinary microscope but can often be seen with a special, high-power microscope. They are considered either very simple microscopic organisms or very complicated *molecules* and can grow and multiply only in living *cells*. They are an important cause of diseases in plants and animals (including you!).

White blood cells: blood *cells* that lack *hemoglobin* but are an important part of the immune system, which helps you to fight off infections. When they do this important work, they cause *inflammation*.

REFERENCES
Definitions and etymologies are derived from the Oxford English Dictionary and Merriam-Webster Dictionary.

Dr. Steven Clark Cunningham
Author

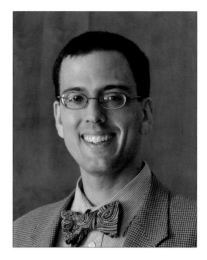

Dr. Steven Clark Cunningham was born in Denver, Colorado. After graduating from Creighton University with majors in chemistry and Spanish, he attended medical school at George Washington University in Washington, DC. Having finished his residency in general surgery at the University of Maryland and a fellowship in surgery of the liver and pancreas at Johns Hopkins University, he currently works as Director of Pancreatic and Hepatobiliary Surgery and Director of Research at Saint Agnes Hospital in Baltimore, MD.

He has served as a contributing editor of *Maryland Poetry Review* and his poems have appeared in that journal. In addition, his work won the literary arts contest sponsored by the magazine *The New Physician*. His poems have also appeared in *Chimeras*, *WordHouse Baltimore's Literary Calendar*, and in the anthologies *Function at the Junction #2*, *Pasta Poetics*, and *Poems for Chromosomes*.

Dinosaur Name Poems (Three Conditions Press, 2009), his first full-length book of children's poetry, won the 2009 Moonbeam Award in both the Children's Poetry and the Spanish Language categories. *Your Body Sick and Well: How Do You Know?* continues to make science fun for kids!

Susan Detwiler
Illustrator

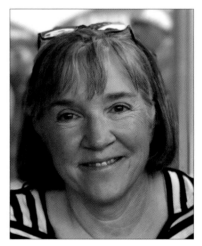

Susan Detwiler has illustrated several award-winning books for children, including *After a While Crocodile*, her sixth title for Arbordale Publishing. She is the author/illustrator of *Fine Life For A Country Mouse*, a picture book published by Penguin Random House in 2014. Her illustrations have appeared in the children's magazines *Highlights for Children* and *Ladybug*. Her artwork has been used for puzzles, games, and greeting cards.

Susan was educated at the Maryland Institute College of Art and lives with her artist husband in Baltimore. She is a member of the Society of Children's Book Writers & Illustrators.